Hypothyroid Diet for Beginners

Understanding the Benefits of Hypothyroid Diet

By

Rannoch Onan

Table of Contents

CHAPTER 1

Introduction

The human endocrine system is a complex network of glands that produce and regulate hormones, influencing nearly every vital process in the body. Among these, the thyroid gland plays a pivotal role in maintaining metabolic balance. Hypothyroidism, a condition where the thyroid gland produces insufficient thyroid hormones, stands as a prevalent and impactful disorder affecting millions worldwide. This introduction aims to shed light on the intricacies of hypothyroidism and underscore the critical role that diet assumes in its management.

1.1 Overview of Hypothyroidism

Hypothyroidism is a thyroid disorder characterized by an underactive thyroid gland, resulting in a reduced production of thyroid hormones, primarily thyroxine (T4) and triiodothyronine (T3). These hormones play a central role in regulating metabolism, energy production, and the functioning of various organs and systems in the body. When the thyroid gland fails to produce an adequate amount of these hormones, it can lead to a range of symptoms such as fatigue, weight gain, sensitivity to cold, and cognitive issues.

The causes of hypothyroidism are diverse, ranging from autoimmune disorders like Hashimoto's thyroiditis to iodine deficiency, medication side effects, or congenital factors. Understanding the root cause is crucial for tailoring effective treatment plans. Additionally, hypothyroidism can manifest at any age, affecting both men and women, although it is more common in women, particularly as they age.

It is paramount to recognize the impact of hypothyroidism on overall health. The condition can extend its influence beyond the thyroid gland, affecting the cardiovascular system, reproductive health, and mental well-being. As such, a comprehensive approach to its management involves not only addressing the hormonal imbalance but also adopting lifestyle and dietary modifications.

1.2 Importance of Diet in Managing Hypothyroidism

The significance of diet in managing hypothyroidism cannot be overstated. The nutrients we consume play a pivotal role in supporting thyroid function and maintaining hormonal balance. Iodine, an essential component of thyroid hormones, is a prime example. A deficiency in iodine can exacerbate hypothyroidism, emphasizing the importance of incorporating iodine-rich foods into the diet.

The interplay between selenium and thyroid health is noteworthy. Selenium acts as a cofactor for enzymes involved in the conversion of T4 to the more active T3 hormone. Thus, ensuring an adequate intake of selenium through dietary sources or supplements can contribute to optimal thyroid function.

The concept of goitrogens, substances that can interfere with thyroid function, adds another layer to the dietary considerations for hypothyroid individuals. Cruciferous vegetables, such as broccoli and cabbage, contain goitrogens and might need moderation in the diet.

Balancing macronutrients, emphasizing whole foods, and avoiding excessive intake of processed sugars and refined carbohydrates are essential components of a hypothyroid-friendly diet. Moreover, understanding the potential interactions between certain medications and dietary components is crucial for individuals managing hypothyroidism.

In essence, a well-crafted diet plan can complement medical interventions, potentially alleviating symptoms and optimizing the management of hypothyroidism. It is not merely about restricting certain foods but about embracing a holistic approach that nourishes the body and supports thyroid health.

CHAPTER 2

Understanding Hypothyroidism

Hypothyroidism is a multifaceted endocrine disorder with a spectrum of causes, varied symptoms, and a need for precise diagnosis and ongoing monitoring. This section delves into the intricacies of hypothyroidism, breaking down its causes, the potential risk factors, the array of symptoms it manifests, and the crucial aspects of its diagnosis and monitoring.

2.1 Causes and Risk Factors

Understanding the root causes of hypothyroidism is pivotal for tailoring effective treatment strategies. The primary cause often lies in the malfunction of the thyroid gland itself. Autoimmune disorders, particularly Hashimoto's thyroiditis, where the body's immune system attacks the thyroid tissue, are leading causes. Other causes include congenital factors, radiation therapy, certain medications (e.g., lithium, amiodarone), and iodine deficiency.

Risk factors for developing hypothyroidism encompass age, with an increased prevalence in older individuals, gender (more common in women), family history of thyroid disorders, and certain medical treatments. Pregnancy can also trigger hypothyroidism, emphasizing the need for prenatal monitoring and care.

2.2 Symptoms of Hypothyroidism

The symptoms of hypothyroidism are diverse and can affect various systems within the body. Understanding these symptoms is crucial for prompt recognition and intervention. Common symptoms include:

- **Fatigue:** Persistent tiredness and lethargy, often unrelieved by sleep.

- **Weight Gain:** Unexplained weight gain despite maintaining a regular diet and exercise routine.

- **Cold Sensitivity:** Intolerance to cold temperatures, with a constant feeling of chilliness.

- **Cognitive Impairment:** Difficulty concentrating, memory issues, and mental fog.

- **Dry Skin and Hair:** Dry, flaky skin and brittle hair are common manifestations.

- **Muscle and Joint Pain:** Aching muscles and joints, often accompanied by stiffness.

- **Menstrual Irregularities:** Changes in menstrual cycle, including heavier or irregular periods.

- **Depression:** Mood changes, including feelings of sadness and depression.

Recognizing these symptoms and their subtle variations is essential for early intervention and effective management.

2.3 Diagnosis and Monitoring

Accurate diagnosis is fundamental for initiating appropriate treatment. Diagnosis involves a combination of clinical evaluation, thyroid function tests measuring levels of TSH (Thyroid Stimulating Hormone), T4, and T3, and imaging studies such as thyroid ultrasound.

Monitoring is an ongoing process, particularly as treatment plans are implemented. Regular thyroid function tests are conducted to assess the effectiveness of medication (commonly synthetic thyroid hormones like levothyroxine), ensuring that hormone levels are within the optimal range. Fine-tuning medication dosage may be necessary to address individual variations in response.

It is imperative for individuals with hypothyroidism to actively participate in their healthcare journey. Understanding the causes, recognizing symptoms, and collaborating with healthcare professionals for accurate diagnosis and continuous monitoring empowers individuals to manage their condition effectively.

CHAPTER 3

Nutrients Essential for Thyroid Health

The optimal functioning of the thyroid gland relies heavily on a balance of specific nutrients. In this section, we delve into the importance of iodine, a crucial element for thyroid health, and explore various dietary sources that can help maintain adequate iodine levels.

3.1 Iodine: Importance and Dietary Sources

Iodine stands as a cornerstone element in the synthesis of thyroid hormones—thyroxine (T4) and triiodothyronine (T3). These hormones play a central role in regulating metabolism, energy production, and the proper functioning of various organs. Iodine deficiency can lead to hypothyroidism, making it essential to understand the significance of iodine and incorporate it into one's diet appropriately.

Importance of Iodine:

1. **Thyroid Hormone Synthesis:** Iodine is an integral component of thyroid hormones. T4 contains four iodine atoms, and T3 contains three. Without sufficient iodine, the thyroid gland cannot produce these hormones in adequate amounts.

2. **Metabolic Regulation:** Thyroid hormones influence

the body's metabolic rate. Adequate iodine levels are essential for maintaining a balanced metabolism, ensuring the efficient conversion of food into energy.

3. **Brain Development:** Iodine is particularly critical during pregnancy and infancy for proper brain development. Severe iodine deficiency during these periods can lead to intellectual disabilities and developmental delays.

Dietary Sources of Iodine:

1. **Seafood:** Seafood, especially fish and shellfish, is a rich source of iodine. Varieties like cod, tuna, shrimp, and seaweed are particularly iodine-rich.

2. **Dairy Products:** Dairy, including milk, cheese, and yogurt, contains iodine. The iodine content varies depending on factors such as the cow's diet and the iodine content in the soil.

3. **Iodized Salt:** Many countries add iodine to table salt to address iodine deficiency. Using iodized salt in cooking and meal preparation is an easy way to ensure sufficient iodine intake.

4. **Eggs:** Eggs, especially those from chickens fed an iodine-rich diet, can contribute to iodine intake.

5. **Iodine Supplements:** In cases where dietary sources may be insufficient, iodine supplements

can be considered. However, it is crucial to consult with a healthcare professional before taking supplements, as excessive iodine intake can also lead to thyroid dysfunction.

Factors Affecting Iodine Levels:

1. **Geographical Location:** The iodine content in soil varies geographically. Regions with iodine-deficient soil may have lower iodine levels in locally grown food.

2. **Dietary Choices:** Individuals adhering to specific diets, such as vegetarian or vegan diets, may need to be mindful of iodine intake, as plant-based sources are generally less rich in iodine.

3. **Pregnancy and Lactation:**
   The iodine requirements
   increase during pregnancy and
   lactation, emphasizing the
   importance of monitoring and
   potentially adjusting iodine
   intake during these periods.

Iodine is a fundamental nutrient for thyroid health, and a well-balanced diet that includes iodine-rich foods is vital for preventing iodine deficiency and maintaining optimal thyroid function. As we navigate through this guide, we will explore other essential nutrients and their roles in supporting overall thyroid health.

3.2 Selenium: Role in Thyroid Function

Selenium and Thyroid Health:

Selenium is an essential mineral that acts as a cofactor for enzymes involved in the conversion of thyroid hormones. One of the key enzymes, known as iodothyronine deiodinase, plays a critical role in the conversion of the inactive thyroid hormone thyroxine (T4) to the active form triiodothyronine (T3). T3 is the form of thyroid hormone that exerts the majority of the biological effects in the body.

The importance of selenium in thyroid function is underscored by its presence in selenoproteins, a family of proteins that includes the deiodinase enzymes. These enzymes are responsible for regulating the levels of T3 and T4, ensuring a finely tuned balance of thyroid hormones in the body.

*Selenium Deficiency and Thyroid
Dysfunction:*

Insufficient selenium levels can lead
to disruptions in the normal
functioning of the thyroid gland.
Selenium deficiency may contribute
to the development or exacerbation of
certain thyroid conditions, including
autoimmune thyroid disorders such as
Hashimoto's thyroiditis and Graves'
disease.

In autoimmune thyroiditis, the
immune system mistakenly attacks
the thyroid gland. Adequate selenium
levels have been associated with a
reduction in antibodies that target the
thyroid, potentially mitigating the
autoimmune response.

Selenium-Rich Foods:

1. **Brazil Nuts:** These nuts are
   exceptionally rich in selenium.

However, consumption should be moderate, as selenium toxicity can occur with excessive intake.

2. **Fish:** Certain fish, such as tuna, halibut, and sardines, are good sources of selenium.

3. **Meat and Poultry:** Beef, chicken, and turkey are selenium-rich meat sources.

4. **Eggs:** Eggs, especially the yolks, contain selenium.

5. **Whole Grains:** Foods like brown rice and whole wheat bread contribute to selenium intake.

6. **Dairy Products:** Milk and yogurt are additional sources of selenium.

Balancing Selenium Intake:

While selenium is crucial for thyroid health, it's equally important to maintain a balance. Too little selenium can lead to deficiencies, while excessive intake can result in toxicity. The recommended daily intake varies by age, sex, and life stage, and it's advisable to obtain selenium through a varied and balanced diet.

Consultation with Healthcare Professionals:

Individuals with thyroid disorders or those considering selenium supplements should consult with healthcare professionals before making significant changes to their diet or taking supplements. The interaction between selenium and thyroid health is intricate, and personalized advice ensures that interventions align with individual health needs.

As we proceed with this comprehensive guide, we will continue to explore additional nutrients, dietary considerations, and lifestyle factors that contribute to the maintenance of optimal thyroid function.

3.3 Zinc, Iron, and Other Trace Minerals

Zinc and Thyroid Function:

Zinc is an essential trace element that participates in various physiological processes, including thyroid hormone metabolism. It plays a crucial role in the synthesis and secretion of thyroid hormones. Zinc deficiency can potentially impair the conversion of T4 to the more active T3 hormone.

Dietary Sources of Zinc:

1. **Meat:** Red meat, poultry, and seafood are rich sources of zinc.

2. **Nuts and Seeds:** Pumpkin seeds, cashews, and almonds contain zinc.

3. **Dairy Products:** Cheese and yogurt provide zinc.

4. **Legumes:** Lentils and chickpeas are plant-based sources of zinc.

Iron and Thyroid Health:

Iron is essential for the proper functioning of the thyroid gland and the production of thyroid hormones. Iron deficiency, commonly known as anemia, can impact thyroid function and contribute to hypothyroidism. On the other hand, excessive iron levels may pose a risk, emphasizing the importance of maintaining a balance.

Dietary Sources of Iron:

1. **Lean Meats:** Beef, pork, and lamb are excellent sources of heme iron, which is more easily absorbed by the body.

2. **Poultry:** Chicken and turkey provide heme iron.

3. **Fish:** Certain fish, such as tuna and salmon, contain iron.

4. **Plant-Based Sources:** Legumes, tofu, and fortified cereals offer non-heme iron, suitable for individuals following vegetarian or vegan diets.

Other Trace Minerals:

1. **Copper:** While required in small amounts, copper is essential for thyroid function. It plays a role in the synthesis of thyroid hormones.

2. **Manganese:** Manganese is involved in the synthesis of thyroxine, a key thyroid hormone.

3. **Sodium and Potassium:** These electrolytes play a role in maintaining the balance of fluids in the body, influencing thyroid function indirectly.

4. **Magnesium:** Magnesium is involved in the conversion of T4 to T3, contributing to the activation of thyroid hormones.

Balancing Trace Minerals:

Achieving a balance of trace minerals is essential for overall health and thyroid function. A diverse and balanced diet that includes a variety of nutrient-rich foods provides the necessary minerals for optimal thyroid health.

Individuals with specific health conditions, dietary restrictions, or concerns about trace mineral intake should consult with healthcare professionals. Nutrient requirements can vary, and personalized advice ensures that dietary choices align with individual health needs.

3.4 Vitamins A, D, and B Complex

Vitamin A and Thyroid Function:

Vitamin A is essential for various physiological processes, including the regulation of thyroid function. It plays a role in supporting the synthesis of thyroid hormones and helps maintain the health of thyroid tissues. Adequate vitamin A levels are essential for optimal thyroid function.

Dietary Sources of Vitamin A:

1. **Liver:** Animal liver, especially from sources like beef and chicken, is a rich source of vitamin A.

2. **Dairy Products:** Milk, cheese, and yogurt contain vitamin A.

3. **Eggs:** Egg yolks provide vitamin A.

4. **Orange and Yellow Vegetables:** Carrots, sweet potatoes, and butternut squash

are rich in beta-carotene, a precursor to vitamin A.

Vitamin D and Thyroid Health:

Vitamin D is crucial for overall health, and its role in supporting the immune system and reducing inflammation is particularly relevant to thyroid health. Additionally, vitamin D receptors are present in thyroid cells, highlighting its importance in thyroid function.

Sources of Vitamin D:

1. **Sun Exposure:** The skin produces vitamin D when exposed to sunlight. Spending time outdoors, especially during midday, contributes to vitamin D synthesis.

2. **Fatty Fish:** Salmon, mackerel, and tuna are excellent sources of vitamin D.

3. **Egg Yolks:** Egg yolks contain vitamin D.

4. **Fortified Foods:** Some foods, such as fortified milk, orange juice, and cereals, are enriched with vitamin D.

B Complex Vitamins and Thyroid Health:

The B complex vitamins, including B1 (thiamine), B2 (riboflavin), B3 (niacin), B6 (pyridoxine), B9 (folate), and B12 (cobalamin), play diverse roles in the body, including supporting energy metabolism and the synthesis of neurotransmitters.

Sources of B Complex Vitamins:

1. **Whole Grains:** B vitamins are abundant in whole grains such as brown rice, oats, and quinoa.

2. **Leafy Greens:** Spinach, kale, and other leafy greens provide various B vitamins.

3. **Meat and Poultry:** Lean meats, poultry, and fish are good sources of B complex vitamins.

4. **Legumes:** Beans and lentils contribute to B vitamin intake.

5. **Dairy Products:** Milk, cheese, and yogurt contain B vitamins.

Balancing Vitamin Intake:

Maintaining a balanced intake of vitamins is essential for overall health and thyroid function. A well-rounded diet that includes a variety of fruits, vegetables, whole grains, lean proteins, and dairy products can contribute to meeting vitamin requirements.

Individuals with specific health conditions, dietary restrictions, or concerns about vitamin intake should consult with healthcare professionals. Personalized advice ensures that dietary choices align with individual health needs.

CHAPTER 4

Impact of Diet

4.1 Impact of Diet on Thyroid Function

Iodine and Thyroid Health:

Iodine is pivotal for thyroid hormone production. Inadequate iodine can lead to hypothyroidism, especially in regions with iodine-deficient diets. However, excessive iodine intake can also disrupt thyroid function.

Selenium's Crucial Role:

Selenium is another micronutrient vital for thyroid health. It aids in the conversion of inactive thyroid hormone (T4) to its active form (T3) and protects the thyroid gland from oxidative damage.

Goitrogens and their Effects:

Goitrogens, present in certain foods like cruciferous vegetables (e.g., broccoli, cabbage), soy, and millet, can interfere with thyroid hormone production if consumed excessively. However, cooking these foods can often neutralize their goitrogenic effects.

Impact of Macronutrients:

Balancing macronutrients—proteins, fats, and carbohydrates—is essential. Low-carb diets might impact thyroid function due to their influence on hormone conversion.

Gluten Sensitivity and Thyroid Health:

Some individuals with hypothyroidism also have gluten sensitivity or celiac disease. Gluten avoidance might aid in managing thyroid function in these cases.

4.2 Common Dietary Mistakes for Hypothyroid Patients

Excessive Intake of Goitrogenic Foods:

Consuming large amounts of raw cruciferous vegetables or soy products can exacerbate hypothyroidism. Cooking these foods reduces their goitrogenic properties.

Inadequate Iodine Consumption:

In regions with low iodine availability, inadequate intake of iodine-rich foods or salt can lead to hypothyroidism. Balancing iodine intake is crucial.

Unbalanced Macronutrient Intake:

Diets overly focused on one macronutrient (e.g., extreme low-carb or high-fat diets) might affect thyroid hormone production and conversion.

Ignoring Nutrient-Dense Foods:

Neglecting foods rich in essential nutrients like selenium, zinc, and iron can impact thyroid function. A diet lacking in variety might lead to nutrient deficiencies.

Not Considering Food Sensitivities:

Individuals with hypothyroidism might have sensitivities to certain foods (like gluten). Ignoring these sensitivities could hinder optimal thyroid health.

Understanding the delicate interplay between diet and hypothyroidism is crucial for managing the condition. Tailoring one's diet to include thyroid-supportive nutrients while avoiding potential triggers can significantly impact thyroid function and overall well-being for those with hypothyroidism. Consulting a healthcare professional or registered dietitian is key in devising a personalized dietary approach to support thyroid health.

CHAPTER 5

Recommended Foods for Hypothyroidism

5.1 Thyroid-Friendly Vegetables

Cruciferous Vegetables:

While often cautioned against due to their goitrogenic properties, cruciferous vegetables like broccoli, Brussels sprouts, kale, and cauliflower can be consumed in moderation when cooked. Cooking these vegetables can help reduce their goitrogenic effects, making them safe for individuals with hypothyroidism.

Spinach and Other Leafy Greens:

Rich in vitamins, minerals, and antioxidants, leafy greens like spinach, Swiss chard, and kale offer a host of nutrients beneficial for thyroid health. These greens are also generally low in goitrogens when compared to cruciferous vegetables.

Bell Peppers:

Colorful bell peppers, especially red and yellow varieties, are excellent sources of vitamin C and antioxidants. Vitamin C supports immune function and aids in the absorption of iron, which is essential for individuals with hypothyroidism.

Carrots and Sweet Potatoes:

These root vegetables are rich in beta-carotene, which the body converts into vitamin A. Vitamin A is crucial for thyroid hormone synthesis and supports overall immune function.

Mushrooms:

Mushrooms are a source of selenium, a mineral important for thyroid health. They also contain antioxidants and are a flavorful addition to various dishes.

Sea Vegetables:

Seaweeds like nori, kombu, and wakame are rich in iodine, a key component of thyroid hormones. However, their iodine content can vary significantly, so portion control is essential to prevent excessive iodine intake.

Onions and Garlic:

These aromatic vegetables contain sulfur compounds that support liver function. The liver plays a role in converting inactive thyroid hormone (T4) to its active form (T3).

When incorporating these thyroid-friendly vegetables into a diet for hypothyroidism, it's important to maintain a balanced and varied intake. Cooking methods that retain nutrients while minimizing goitrogenic effects, such as steaming or sautéing, can be beneficial.

5.2 Lean Proteins and Hypothyroidism

Poultry (Chicken, Turkey):

Lean cuts of poultry are excellent sources of high-quality protein. They also provide essential amino acids necessary for various bodily functions, including thyroid hormone production.

Fish:

Fatty fish like salmon, mackerel, sardines, and trout are rich in omega-3 fatty acids. Omega-3s have anti-inflammatory properties and support overall thyroid health. Additionally, fish is a good source of selenium, which plays a role in thyroid hormone metabolism.

Legumes and Beans:

Plant-based sources of protein like lentils, chickpeas, and black beans are not only protein-rich but also provide fiber and essential nutrients. They are suitable alternatives for individuals following a vegetarian or vegan diet.

Lean Cuts of Red Meat:

Lean beef, pork tenderloin, and lean cuts of lamb provide high-quality protein and essential nutrients like iron and zinc. Iron is particularly important for individuals with hypothyroidism as deficiency can exacerbate symptoms.

5.3 Healthy Fats for Thyroid Health

Avocado:

Rich in monounsaturated fats, avocados also provide essential nutrients like potassium and vitamins E and K. These fats support heart health and may aid in reducing inflammation.

Nuts and Seeds:

Almonds, walnuts, chia seeds, and flaxseeds are excellent sources of healthy fats, including omega-3 fatty acids. They also offer a range of

vitamins and minerals beneficial for
overall health.

Olive Oil:

Extra virgin olive oil contains
monounsaturated fats and
antioxidants, offering numerous
health benefits, including potential
anti-inflammatory effects.

Coconut Oil:

While controversial, some research
suggests that coconut oil, with its
medium-chain triglycerides (MCTs),
may support thyroid function.
However, moderation is key due to its
high saturated fat content.

Fatty Fish:

As mentioned earlier, fatty fish like
salmon and mackerel are not only
excellent sources of protein but also

provide omega-3 fatty acids essential for thyroid health.

Incorporating lean proteins and healthy fats into the diet of someone managing hypothyroidism can help maintain a balanced and nutritious eating plan. It's important to customize the intake based on individual needs and dietary preferences.

5.4 Whole Grains and Fiber

Whole grains and fiber play significant roles in a hypothyroid diet by providing essential nutrients and supporting digestive health. Here's a detailed breakdown of their importance:

Whole Grain Varieties:

- **Quinoa:** Rich in protein and fiber, quinoa is a gluten-free grain that offers a balanced set of amino acids and essential nutrients like iron and magnesium.

- **Brown Rice:** A nutritious whole grain that provides fiber, B vitamins, and minerals like selenium and magnesium, important for thyroid health.

- **Oats:** High in soluble fiber, oats support digestive health and can help regulate cholesterol levels.

Fiber-Rich Foods:

- **Legumes:** Beans, lentils, and chickpeas are excellent sources of fiber, aiding in digestion and promoting a healthy gut microbiome.

- **Fruits and Vegetables:**
  Berries, apples, pears, and
  vegetables like broccoli and
  Brussels sprouts provide fiber
  along with vitamins, minerals,
  and antioxidants.

Importance of Fiber for
Hypothyroidism:

- **Regulating Bowel
  Movements:** Constipation is a
  common symptom of
  hypothyroidism, and fiber helps
  alleviate this issue by
  promoting regular bowel
  movements.

- **Supporting Gut Health:** A
  healthy gut microbiome is
  linked to improved overall
  health, including better immune
  function and potential positive
  effects on thyroid health.

- **Balancing Blood Sugar Levels:** Fiber slows down the absorption of sugar, aiding in stabilizing blood sugar levels, which can fluctuate in individuals with hypothyroidism.

Considerations for Gluten Sensitivity:

- Some individuals with hypothyroidism might also have gluten sensitivity. For them, opting for gluten-free whole grains like quinoa, rice, and gluten-free oats might be more suitable.

Preparation Methods:

- Soaking, sprouting, or fermenting grains and legumes before consumption can help break down anti-nutrients and enhance nutrient absorption.

When incorporating whole grains and fiber into a hypothyroid diet, it's crucial to maintain variety and monitor how the body responds to different sources. Moderation and balance are key, as excessive fiber intake might affect the absorption of certain medications commonly prescribed for hypothyroidism.

CHAPTER 6

Foods to Limit or Avoid

6.1 Goitrogenic Foods and Their Effects

What are Goitrogens?

- Goitrogens are compounds found in certain foods that can interfere with the normal function of the thyroid gland by potentially blocking the uptake of iodine or inhibiting thyroid hormone production.

Common Goitrogenic Foods:

1. **Cruciferous Vegetables:** Broccoli, cabbage, cauliflower, kale, Brussels sprouts, and bok

choy are among the most notable. Cooking these vegetables often reduces their goitrogenic properties.

2. **Soy-Based Products:** Soybeans, tofu, soy milk, and edamame contain goitrogens. Fermented soy products like miso or tempeh tend to have lower goitrogenic effects.

3. **Millets:** Certain grains like millet, if consumed in large amounts, may have goitrogenic effects.

Effects of Goitrogenic Foods:

- **Interference with Iodine Absorption:** Goitrogens might hinder the body's ability to absorb iodine, an essential element for thyroid hormone production. In iodine-deficient areas, this interference could exacerbate hypothyroidism.

- **Thyroid Hormone Disruption:** In some cases, excessive consumption of goitrogenic foods might interfere with the production or conversion of thyroid hormones, impacting thyroid function.

Moderation and Preparation:

- **Cooking Methods:** Cooking goitrogenic foods can often neutralize or reduce their goitrogenic effects. For instance, steaming or boiling cruciferous vegetables can make them safer for consumption.

- **Portion Control:** It's important to consume these foods in moderation, especially if you have an existing thyroid condition or are sensitive to goitrogens.

Individual Sensitivities:

- **Variability in Effects:** Not everyone with hypothyroidism is equally sensitive to goitrogens. Some individuals may tolerate these foods without any noticeable impact on thyroid function.

- **Personal Observation:** Monitoring how your body reacts to certain goitrogenic foods can help identify any adverse effects on thyroid health. Keeping a food diary might assist in understanding individual tolerances.

While goitrogenic foods have the potential to affect thyroid function, their impact varies among individuals. For most people, incorporating these foods in moderate amounts, particularly when cooked, is unlikely to cause significant issues. However, those with specific sensitivities or concerns should consider consulting a healthcare provider or a registered dietitian for personalized guidance regarding their diet and managing hypothyroidism.

6.2 Processed Foods and Sugars

Processed Foods:

- **Highly Processed Items:** Foods high in refined sugars, artificial additives, preservatives, and trans fats should be limited. These include fast food, sugary snacks, processed meats, and certain packaged foods.

Impact of Processed Foods:

- **Inflammatory Response:** Highly processed foods can trigger inflammation in the body, potentially exacerbating autoimmune conditions often associated with hypothyroidism, such as Hashimoto's thyroiditis.

- **Nutrient Deficiency:** Processed foods are often low in essential nutrients and high in empty calories, contributing to potential nutrient deficiencies that can affect thyroid health.

Refined Sugars:

- **Blood Sugar Imbalances:** Refined sugars found in candies, pastries, sugary beverages, and many processed foods can cause rapid spikes and crashes in blood sugar levels, which may impact hormone regulation, including thyroid hormones.

- **Inflammation:** Excessive sugar consumption has been linked to increased inflammation in the body, which might negatively impact thyroid function and exacerbate symptoms of hypothyroidism.

6.3 Potential Allergens and Sensitivities

Common Allergens:

- **Gluten:** Some individuals with hypothyroidism may have gluten sensitivity or celiac disease, and gluten consumption can potentially trigger autoimmune responses affecting the thyroid.

- **Dairy:** Sensitivity to dairy products might aggravate inflammation for some individuals, impacting thyroid function. Substituting dairy with non-dairy alternatives might be beneficial.

Effects on the Gut:

- **Gut Health:** Allergens or sensitivities can affect gut health, potentially leading to intestinal permeability ("leaky gut"), which has been associated with autoimmune conditions, including some forms of hypothyroidism.

Personalized Approach:

- **Identifying Triggers:** Keeping a food diary and noting any adverse reactions or changes in symptoms after consuming certain foods can help identify potential allergens or sensitivities.

- **Elimination Diets:** Some individuals might benefit from temporary elimination diets to identify trigger foods and alleviate symptoms associated with food sensitivities.

Taking steps to limit processed foods, refined sugars, and potential allergens or sensitivities can contribute to managing inflammation, supporting gut health, and potentially alleviating symptoms associated with hypothyroidism. However, it's essential to approach dietary changes cautiously and seek guidance from a healthcare provider or a registered dietitian, especially when considering elimination diets or making significant alterations to one's diet, to ensure nutritional adequacy and proper management of the condition.

CHAPTER 7

Meal Planning for Hypothyroid Individuals

meal planning for individuals with hypothyroidism involves balancing macronutrients and creating nutrient-rich meals to support overall health and manage the condition effectively:

7.1 Balancing Macronutrients

Importance of Macronutrients:

- **Proteins:** Essential for tissue repair, hormone production, and supporting a healthy metabolism. Opt for lean proteins like poultry, fish, legumes, and nuts.

- **Carbohydrates:** Focus on complex carbohydrates from whole grains, fruits, and vegetables to provide sustained energy and fiber while avoiding rapid blood sugar spikes.

- **Fats:** Prioritize healthy fats like those found in avocados, nuts, seeds, and fatty fish. These fats support hormone production and assist in nutrient absorption.

Individualized Needs:

- **Customizing Ratios:** Balancing macronutrients should be tailored to individual needs and tolerances. Some individuals might benefit from a higher protein or fat intake depending on their overall health and activity levels.

- **Monitoring Responses:** Observing how the body responds to different macronutrient ratios can help fine-tune a meal plan that best supports energy levels and overall well-being.

7.2 Creating Nutrient-Rich Meals

Emphasis on Nutrient Density:

- **Variety of Whole Foods:** Include a diverse range of vegetables, fruits, whole grains, lean proteins, and healthy fats in each meal to maximize nutrient intake.

- **Colorful Plate:** Aim for a colorful plate, incorporating different fruits and vegetables of various hues to ensure a broad spectrum of vitamins, minerals, and antioxidants.

Key Nutrients for Thyroid Health:

- **Iodine:** Incorporate iodine-rich foods like seaweed, fish, dairy (if tolerated), and iodized salt in moderation to support thyroid function.

- **Selenium:** Include selenium sources such as Brazil nuts, seafood, poultry, and whole grains to aid in thyroid hormone conversion.

Meal Planning Tips:

- **Portion Control:** Balance portion sizes to avoid

overconsumption, especially of goitrogenic foods, and maintain a well-rounded diet.

- **Regular Eating Schedule:** Aim for regular, balanced meals throughout the day to maintain stable energy levels and support metabolic function.

Sample Nutrient-Rich Meals:

- **Breakfast:** Greek yogurt with berries and nuts or oatmeal with seeds, fruit, and a sprinkle of cinnamon.

- **Lunch:** Grilled chicken salad with mixed greens, colorful veggies, quinoa, and an olive oil-based dressing.

- **Dinner:** Baked salmon with roasted sweet potatoes and a side of steamed broccoli or stir-fried tofu with vegetables and brown rice.

Tailoring meals to include a variety of nutrient-dense foods while balancing macronutrients is key for individuals managing hypothyroidism. This approach supports overall health, provides essential nutrients for thyroid function, and helps manage energy levels throughout the day.

7.3 Sample Meal Plans

Here are sample meal plans tailored for individuals managing hypothyroidism:

Sample Meal Plan 1:

Day 1:

- **Breakfast:** Greek yogurt parfait with mixed berries, chia seeds, and a drizzle of honey.

- **Lunch:** Quinoa salad with mixed vegetables (bell peppers, cucumber, spinach) and grilled chicken.

- **Dinner:** Baked salmon fillet with roasted sweet potatoes and steamed broccoli.

Day 2:

- **Breakfast:** Spinach and feta omelet with a side of whole-grain toast.

- **Lunch:** Lentil soup with a side of mixed green salad and vinaigrette dressing.

- **Dinner:** Stir-fried tofu with colorful bell peppers, snap peas, and brown rice.

Day 3:

- **Breakfast:** Overnight oats made with almond milk, topped with sliced bananas and almonds.

- **Lunch:** Turkey and avocado wrap with whole-grain tortilla, accompanied by carrot sticks.

- **Dinner:** Grilled chicken breast with quinoa pilaf and roasted Brussels sprouts.

Sample Meal Plan 2:

Day 1:

- **Breakfast:** Smoothie made with spinach, banana, almond milk, and a scoop of protein powder.

- **Lunch:** Mixed greens salad with grilled shrimp, cherry

tomatoes, and a sprinkle of pumpkin seeds.

- **Dinner:** Baked cod with a side of steamed asparagus and wild rice.

Day 2:

- **Breakfast:** Whole-grain toast topped with mashed avocado and poached eggs.

- **Lunch:** Chickpea salad with cucumbers, tomatoes, feta cheese, and a lemon-tahini dressing.

- **Dinner:** Vegetable stir-fry with tofu, served over quinoa.

Day 3:

- **Breakfast:** Greek yogurt bowl with sliced peaches, a handful of granola, and a drizzle of honey.

- **Lunch:** Whole-grain wrap filled with hummus, roasted vegetables, and grilled chicken.

- **Dinner:** Baked turkey meatballs with zucchini noodles and marinara sauce.

These sample meal plans offer variety and include nutrient-dense foods that support thyroid health while providing balanced macronutrients. Adjusting portion sizes and specific food choices according to individual preferences and dietary needs can further personalize these meal plans.

CHAPTER 8

Cooking and Preparation Tips

Here are cooking and preparation tips specifically catered to retain nutrients and flavor while maintaining a health-conscious approach:

8.1 Cooking Methods for Retaining Nutrients

Steaming:

- **Benefits:** Steaming vegetables helps retain their nutrients by cooking them quickly in steam rather than boiling in water, which can leach out vitamins and minerals.

- **Usage:** Use a steamer basket or a steaming rack over boiling water to cook vegetables until they are tender yet still vibrant in color.

Sautéing and Stir-Frying:

- **Benefits:** Cooking quickly over high heat in a small amount of oil preserves nutrients and enhances flavor. Use heart-healthy oils like olive oil or avocado oil.

- **Usage:** Cut vegetables or lean proteins into small, uniform pieces for even cooking and to retain their nutrients.

Roasting or Baking:

- **Benefits:** Roasting or baking vegetables caramelizes their natural sugars, enhancing taste while preserving nutrients.

- **Usage:** Use a moderate oven temperature and a light coating of healthy oil. Avoid overcooking to maintain nutrient content.

Lightly Cooking Greens:

- **Benefits:** Quickly blanching or lightly cooking greens like spinach or kale can soften them without significant nutrient loss.

- **Usage:** Plunge greens into boiling water for a short time (usually a minute or less) before cooling immediately in ice water to preserve their color and nutrients.

8.2 Flavoring Without Compromising Health

Herbs and Spices:

- **Benefits:** Fresh or dried herbs and spices add flavor without added sodium or calories. Incorporate basil, oregano, turmeric, cumin, or cinnamon for added taste and health benefits.

- **Usage:** Experiment with different combinations to enhance the taste of dishes without relying on excessive salt or sugar.

Citrus Juices and Zest:

- **Benefits:** Citrus fruits like lemons, limes, and oranges add a zesty, tangy flavor while providing vitamin C and antioxidants.

- **Usage:** Use zest or freshly squeezed juice to season salads, marinades, or sauces for a burst of flavor.

Natural Umami Ingredients:

- **Benefits:** Umami-rich ingredients like mushrooms, tomatoes, miso, and nutritional yeast add depth and savory flavors to dishes.

- **Usage:** Incorporate these ingredients into soups, stews, or sauces to enhance taste without relying on added salt or unhealthy flavor enhancers.

Homemade Seasoning Blends:

- **Benefits:** Create custom seasoning blends using dried

herbs, spices, and minimal salt to add flavor to meals without compromising health.

- **Usage:** Experiment with combinations such as Italian seasoning, taco seasoning, or curry blends to season various dishes.

By employing these cooking methods and flavoring techniques, individuals managing hypothyroidism can retain the nutritional value of foods while enhancing taste without excessive use of unhealthy additives. Customizing these approaches according to personal preferences can elevate the culinary experience while supporting overall health goals.

CHAPTER 9

Lifestyle Factors and Hypothyroidism

9.1 Importance of Regular Exercise

Benefits of Exercise for Hypothyroidism:

- **Metabolic Boost:** Exercise supports metabolism, aiding in weight management—a common concern for individuals with hypothyroidism.

- **Improved Mood:** Physical activity can enhance mood and alleviate symptoms of depression, which might accompany hypothyroidism.

- **Energy Levels:** Regular exercise can help combat fatigue; a common symptom associated with hypothyroidism.

Exercise Recommendations:

- **Aerobic Activities:** Brisk walking, cycling, swimming, or aerobics can improve cardiovascular health and support weight management.

- **Strength Training:** Incorporating resistance exercises or weight training helps build muscle mass and supports metabolic rate.

Considerations:

- **Moderation:** Individuals with hypothyroidism should start slowly and gradually increase the intensity and duration of exercise to avoid exhaustion or strain.

9.2 Stress Management Techniques

Stress and Hypothyroidism:

- **Impact on Hormones:** Chronic stress can affect hormone levels, potentially worsening symptoms of hypothyroidism.

- **Inflammation:** Stress can trigger inflammation, impacting immune function and potentially exacerbating autoimmune thyroid conditions.

Stress Management Strategies:

- **Mindfulness and Meditation:** Practices like meditation, deep breathing exercises, or yoga can help reduce stress levels and promote relaxation.

- **Regular Physical Activity:** Exercise not only benefits physical health but also helps manage stress and improve mental well-being.

- **Healthy Boundaries and Support:** Establishing healthy boundaries, seeking support from friends or professionals, and practicing time management can reduce stress.

9.3 Sleep and Its Impact on Thyroid Health:

Importance of Quality Sleep:

- **Hormonal Balance:** Quality sleep supports hormonal regulation, including thyroid hormones, aiding in overall metabolic function.

- **Restoration and Healing:** Adequate sleep facilitates the body's repair processes and supports immune function.

- **Impact on Mood and Energy:** Quality sleep contributes to improved mood and sustained energy levels.

Strategies for Better Sleep:

- **Consistent Sleep Schedule:** Aim for a regular sleep routine, going to bed and waking up at the same time each day.

- **Sleep Environment:** Create a comfortable sleep environment, ensuring it is dark, quiet, and conducive to restful sleep.

- **Stress Reduction:** Implement relaxation techniques or practices before bedtime to unwind and prepare the body for sleep.

Prioritizing regular exercise, stress management, and quality sleep are integral components of managing hypothyroidism. Incorporating these lifestyle factors alongside proper medication and dietary strategies can significantly improve overall well-being and assist in managing symptoms associated with the condition.

CHAPTER 10

Consulting a Healthcare Professional

10.1 Importance of Medical Guidance

Proper Diagnosis and Treatment:

- **Accurate Diagnosis:** Healthcare professionals diagnose hypothyroidism through blood tests measuring thyroid hormone levels, ensuring an accurate diagnosis before creating a treatment plan.

- **Medication Management:** Doctors prescribe hormone

replacement therapy (e.g., synthetic thyroid hormone) based on individual needs and monitor its effectiveness through regular check-ups and blood tests.

Monitoring and Adjusting Treatment:

- **Regular Follow-ups:** Healthcare providers monitor thyroid hormone levels, symptoms, and potential side effects of medications, adjusting dosages as needed.

- **Potential Complications:** Regular medical check-ups help detect and address any complications or changes in thyroid function promptly.

10.2 Working with a Registered Dietitian

Personalized Dietary Guidance:

- **Nutritional Assessment:** Registered dietitians assess individual nutritional needs, considering factors like age, gender, activity level, and specific health conditions like hypothyroidism.

- **Tailored Diet Plans:** They design personalized meal plans that align with the individual's dietary preferences while addressing nutritional deficiencies and supporting thyroid health.

Education and Support:

- **Nutritional Education:** Dietitians provide information

on foods rich in essential nutrients for thyroid health and offer guidance on managing goitrogenic foods or potential allergens.

- **Behavioral Changes:** They assist in implementing dietary changes and offer ongoing support to ensure adherence to a hypothyroid-friendly diet.

Collaboration with Healthcare Team:

- **Integrated Approach:** Registered dietitians collaborate with doctors and other healthcare providers to align dietary strategies with medical treatment and overall health management.

Seeking guidance from healthcare professionals ensures a comprehensive and integrated approach to managing hypothyroidism. While doctors oversee medication and treatment, registered dietitians offer crucial dietary support and education, creating personalized meal plans that optimize thyroid health. Collaboration between these professionals allows for a holistic approach, addressing various aspects of the condition to improve overall well-being and quality of life for individuals with hypothyroidism.

www.ingramcontent.com/pod-product-compliance
Lightning Source LLC
Chambersburg PA
CBHW060953260726
48661CB00005B/1870